SIATISM EXERCISES HANDBOOK

EXERCISES FOR SCIATICA AND HOW TO PERFORM THEM

GARRETT MORAN

Table of Contents

CHAPTER ONE

SIATISM EXERCISES

Painful Sciatica? Try These Exercises!

A carefully designed and gradually increased exercise regimen is the gold standard for treating sciatica. The underlying cause of pain is addressed, resolved, and prevented from recurring thanks to the exercise treatment.

The following are some of the most important goals of sciatica-specific exercise:

Lessen the intensity of sudden sciatica pain

Increase flexibility and range of motion in the legs.

• Facilitate the repair of soft tissues

• Revitalize the sciatic nerve's capacity

Intensify muscular and connective tissue conditioning

To: • Avoid or, at the very least, lessen the occurrence of pain flare-ups

Therapeutic exercises are most beneficial when they are performed frequently and as directed, according to the prescribed form and program. It can be difficult to focus on proper form during exercise, but doing so is crucial for achieving the desired results.

The most common causes of pain along the sciatic nerve are addressed in this in-depth guide to therapeutic exercise for sciatica.

Pain from sciatica can be reduced with exercise.

Exercise, contrary to popular belief, is more helpful for relieving sciatica pain than either bed rest or continuing to engage in normal physical activities.

1,2 Prescribed exercise is distinct from regular physical activity in that it is designed to meet specific goals and involves a systematic, progressive process that has been shown to enhance fitness levels. 3

Sciatica pain can be managed with a short period of rest and limited movement, but prolonged inactivity usually makes the condition worse. Sciatica pain relief is a result of the following tissue changes brought on by regular exercise:

The power of your muscles has grown. The activation (correct muscle engagement) and area of deep muscle fibers both increase with exercise, leading to greater muscle strength.

Four, five Muscular strength aids in spinal stability. 6-8 Also alleviated is the discomfort associated with muscle fatigue.

Strengthening of bones is a benefit. Physical activity boosts bone density, which in turn makes your bones stronger. Exercise has been shown to improve bone quality in conditions like osteoporosis and bone pain from arthritis and ankylosing spondylitis. 7,9

It has been shown to improve circulation. The muscles, nerves, and other soft tissues in the spine benefit from an increase in blood flow thanks to regular exercise. This improves blood flow, which helps heal damaged tissues and eases stiffness. 8,10

Benefits to the spinal discs have been nourished. The spinal discs nourish and lubricate the spinal column by passing fluid back and forth between the spinal vertebrae. A healthy disc absorbs fluid and nutrients, then squeezes the excess out like a sponge. Applying forces to the disc during exercise promotes this action by facilitating the transport of nutrients across the disc.

The sciatic nerve's usual stiffness has been diminished. Mobilization and stretching exercises, also known as "nerve glide," can help alleviate sciatic nerve stiffness. These routines keep the nutrients flowing to the nerve and the tissues around it, keeping the nerve supple and healthy. Along with alleviating nerve swelling, this method can also counteract the immune system's dysfunctional shifts.

Back muscles and spinal structures become

deconditioned (weak and stiff) and less able to support the back without regular exercise and movement. When you're out of shape, you're more vulnerable to injuries and strains that can make things hurt even more.

Exercises for Sciatica Aim at the Root of the Pain

When people talk about having sciatica, they're referring to a collection of symptoms rather than a specific medical condition. Sciatic pain is called radiculopathy in the medical field. Herniated or degenerated discs, spinal stenosis, and spondylolisthesis in the lumbar spine are all potential causes of sciatica symptoms.

Typically, sciatica exercises are designed to address the patient's unique etiology. Some common causes of sciatica pain are addressed by a wide variety of exercises, and some examples are provided below.

Abdominal and core strengthening exercises, as well as pain centralization therapy like the McKenzie technique, can help with herniated discs.

Back and hip flexor flexibility is increased and abdominal muscle strength is increased with flexion (forward bending) exercises for spinal stenosis.

• Exercises aimed at strengthening the back and core muscles and reducing excessive micromotions in the disc space may be effective in treating degenerated spinal discs that cause spinal instability and, in turn, leg pain.

To stop the vertebra from slipping forward due to isthmic spondylolisthesis, treatment may involve bolstering the back's core muscles and providing more support for the spine.

CHAPTER TWO

Instructions for Exercising to Ease Sciatica

The following are some of the fundamentals shared by the majority of individualized exercise plans.

Strengthening the abdominal muscles

Exercises for sciatica often focus on strengthening the core muscles (abdominals, back, and pelvic floor) to alleviate pressure on the spine. Patients with a history of sciatica can benefit from a routine of gentle core strengthening exercises, which has been shown to reduce the frequency and severity of pain episodes.

Promoting Hamstring Flexibility

A regular routine of hamstring stretching is helpful for most forms of sciatica. Those muscles at the top of one's thighs are called the hamstrings. Tight hamstrings can aggravate or even cause some of the conditions that lead to sciatica because they increase pressure on the lower back.

Involvement in aerobic exercise

The benefits of aerobic conditioning include improved cardiovascular health, increased blood flow, and the production of endorphins, the body's natural painkillers. Just 30 minutes of walking a day can give you all the health benefits of an intensive aerobic workout. A pleasant and manageable walking pace is possible. Building up to a daily brisk walk of up to three miles is ideal as fitness levels rise.

Maintaining spinal support all day can help lessen sciatica symptoms.

Modifying activities and improving ergonomics in daily life is usually necessary to prevent further sciatic nerve irritation. Some general suggestions are as follows:

Correct lifting posture includes: bending at the knees and leading with the hips

• Keeping a straight back when standing, walking, and sitting

In order to avoid muscle fatigue, you should avoid prolonged periods of standing or sitting.

Propping up one foot on a step stool while standing for extended periods of time

Protect your spinal discs by avoiding bending and twisting first thing in the morning.

The use of heat therapy prior to physical activity or upon waking in the morning can help loosen up stiff muscles and increase spinal flexibility.

Doing light aerobic exercise for 10 minutes as a warmup before more strenuous exercise.

Utilizing an ice pack to lessen muscle soreness after exercise or physical activity

Putting a pillow under your knees if you sleep on your back, or between your legs if you prefer to sleep on your side.

Sciatic nerve pain should be properly diagnosed by a medical professional before any exercise regimen is started. It is important to get a correct diagnosis to rule out more serious conditions like tumors, infections, and cauda equina syndrome. Incorrect self-treatment for sciatica is likely to make the condition worse by irritating the sciatic nerve even more. Exercising properly requires instruction from a qualified instructor and regular participation in a structured program.

Medical Practitioners Who Lead Patients Through Therapeutic Exercise

Physical therapists, physiatrists, certified athletic trainers (ATC), and chiropractors are just some of the healthcare professionals who are qualified to prescribe and instruct patients on therapeutic exercises for the treatment of musculoskeletal disorders of the spine. Depending on the patient's age, the severity of the underlying cause, and/or the patient's level of tolerability, they may also adjust the exercises' intensity and frequency. In order to get the most out of any workout, it is crucial to breathe normally and take breaks as needed. Stop exercising and talk to your therapist if you start to feel any pain or discomfort.

CHAPTER THREE

Corrective moves for sciatica

If you suffer from sciatica, you may find that certain exercises and stretches help alleviate the pain and tightness in your sciatic nerve and the surrounding muscles. Although sciatica usually goes away on its own, doing these exercises may help it go away faster.

Managing the radiating pain of sciatica can be particularly challenging, and it can sometimes even be debilitating. However, resting may not help sciatica pain, unlike many other types of pain.

Several exercises are outlined, along with an explanation of their efficacy in reducing sciatic pain. The article also discusses sciatica's symptoms and signs, as well as ways to avoid getting it and various treatments available.

A set of stretches and exercises numbering seven

A reliable source estimates that most cases of sciatica resolve within four to six weeks. However, it's possible that certain stretches and exercises could aid in the recovery process and decrease discomfort.

The following exercises are designed to improve gluteus, piriformis, hamstring, and lower back strength and flexibility.

Regular practice of these motions is recommended for the best outcomes. But because the sciatic nerve is affected differently by the various causes of sciatica, not everyone will benefit from all of the exercises.

Although stretching and tension are intended effects of exercise, they should not aggravate existing pain or give rise to any new discomfort.

Put your knee up to your chest.

To accomplish this, the following procedures are used:

To do this, lie on your back with your legs bent at the knees and your feet flat on the floor.

One foot should be left flat on the floor while the other knee is pulled to the chest.

Keep the knee close to the chest for as long as you feel comfortable, ideally around 30 seconds.

• When you're ready, slowly let go of the leg and switch to the other one.

Try to complete three sets for each leg. The variation of this stretch involves bringing both legs to the chest and holding the position for 30 seconds.

Leg muscles that connect at the thighs

Those interested in performing glute bridges can do so by following these instructions:

Lay on your back with your knees bent and feet flat on the

floor, about shoulder-width apart.

In order to achieve this, you should drive through the heels and lift the hips until a straight line can be drawn from the shins to the shoulders.

• Remain in this position for as long as you feel comfortable before lowering your hips back to the floor.

Aim for 8 to 10 reps at first, and once that's comfortable, work your way up to multiple sets.

Seated Pigeon Position

There's a good chance that those who regularly practice yoga will recognize this posture change:

• Cross your legs in front of you while sitting on the floor.

What you want to do is cross your right ankle over your left knee while bending your right knee.

In this position, you should stoop forward from the hips and let your upper body fall naturally toward your thigh.

Alternately, if you are able to do so without too much pain, you can increase the stretch by bending your left leg in and placing your hands behind your thigh.

Ten to twenty seconds is ideal, but go with what feels good for you.

Then, after a moment, let go and stretch the other side.

Forward bending while seated

The following exercises can also help people stretch their trunks:

• While seated, extend both legs straight out in front of you and flex your toes upward.

Simply lift your right foot, flex your right knee, and set it on the outside of your left leg, just above the knee.

Position your left elbow outside your right knee and gently push into it as you twist your torso to the right.

You should squeeze for 20-30 seconds, then let go and switch sides.

Do this a few times on each side.

Baby's Pose

The following are the steps to this popular yoga pose:

To begin, get down on your knees and rest your buttocks on your heels.

• Place the body on the floor with the knees about as far apart as the hips.

• Place your arms on the floor in front of your head and rest them there.

• Take a few deep breaths and settle into the posture. Don't try to force your buttocks onto your heels; rather, let them rest there for a few moments to get a nice stretch.

Try to maintain the position for at least 30 seconds before easing out of it.

Hamstring stretches while standing

For this stretch, a low, stable surface is required for the person's foot:

• Maintain an erect stance, with one foot propped up on a low object (a stool or stair step works well) that is higher than the other foot but lower than the hips.

Straighten your leg and flex your foot so that your toes point upward.

To activate the hamstring, lean forward slightly at the hips while bringing the upper body closer to the knee. Keep your spine erect.

• Get as low as you can go without straining, but don't go too low.

Please maintain this position for at least 30 seconds, or as long as is tolerable for you.

Then, ease off and do the same with the other leg.

Two to three sets should be performed on each leg.

Body position characterized by a swaying pelvis

This move helps build strength in the lower back, glutes, and abs:

Position yourself on your back, with your knees bent and your arms at your sides.

• Contract your abs and tuck your chin in, keeping your back flat against the floor.

Pose by lifting the hips and pelvis and holding the position while concentrating on the breath for a few seconds.

Put your foot down and unwind.

Start with 10 reps and increase that number gradually if you can.

CHAPTER FOUR

The British Medical Journal suggests that physical activity be viewed by medical professionals as a primary component of noninvasive treatment.

This is because unlike with some injuries, sciatica pain may get better with exercise rather than rest. Furthermore, keeping up with the exercises even after the pain has subsided may help reduce the likelihood of a recurrence.

The following are some possible contributors to a reduction in sciatica symptoms:

Strengthening of Muscles

Strengthening the surrounding muscles through exercise can help alleviate pressure on the injured structures. Targeted exercises aid in back stabilization and increase mobility, as reported in the

Journal of Exercise Rehabilitation (Reliable Source). By doing so, they may lessen strain on the disks that house the sciatic nerve.

higher blood pressure

The muscles and nerves in the area benefit from increased blood flow thanks to exercise. With better circulation, oxygenated blood can more easily reach the area in need, while waste products and inflammation can be carried away.

Enhanced condition of connective tissues

If you suffer from sciatica, doing regular mobilization exercises may help heal the soft tissues in the disks and keep them healthy. Exercise may promote healthy nutrient and fluid exchange between spinal disks, according to research. Therefore, inactivity and lack of exercise can be detrimental to the disks.

Recovery of Nerve Function

By stimulating the nervous system, specific exercises for sciatica were found to improve nerve health markers, such as stiffness and sensitivity.

Explain the nature of sciatica.

Pain along the sciatic nerve is known as sciatica. The sciatic nerve begins in the lower back, travels through the buttocks, and divides into four separate nerves as it descends each leg. In some spots, the nerve's diameter can reach up to 2 centimeters.

Because of the location of the nerve pinch, sciatica typically only affects one leg and the same side of the body. Pain that spreads outward from the source, possibly all the way to the butt, the back of the leg, or the feet and toes.

There's a chance that the affected region will feel weaker than usual, too. Back pain is a common symptom, but it may seem less significant than the pain radiating from the sciatic nerve.

CHAPTER FIVE

Why do people get sciatica?

When the sciatic nerve becomes aggravated and inflamed, pain is felt down the leg. Nonetheless, there isn't always a clear reason why a person is experiencing sciatica.

When the sciatic nerve is pinched because of a slipped or herniated disk, pain can result. The spinal column is cushioned by disks of cartilage, which also contribute to the spine's pliability.

There are other potential triggers for sciatic pain.

• Spinal infections that have spread

Spinal cord injuries

tumors of the spinal column

The narrowing of the spinal canal, medically known as spinal stenosis

Spondylolisthesis is a condition in which a disk slips over a vertebra.

Symptoms of cauda equina syndrome include weakness in the legs and buttocks and pain radiating up the legs and buttocks.

What measures can be taken to keep people free of sciatica?

The likelihood of developing sciatica or avoiding the back damage that could lead to it can be greatly increased by taking some simple precautions.

Some fundamental precautions are:

Lifting heavy objects safely and correctly

Doing muscle-strengthening exercises on a consistent basis.

• trying not to sit or stand for too long

• not doing anything that could cause pain, like bending or twisting, until you've warmed up

• taking a few minutes to limber up before getting to work

Is there any other kind of treatment available?

Home remedies and anti-inflammatory drugs are also options for treating sciatica.

Therapeutic Medicine

The following medications are often suggested or prescribed by doctors for the treatment of sciatica:

drugs that reduce inflammation but aren't NSAIDs

Calming Agents for Muscles

• anticonvulsants

Subcutaneous injections of corticosteroids

Common treatments

To alleviate sciatica symptoms at home, try:

To alleviate pain and swelling, heat and cold packs can be used.

- committing to a regular routine of light exercise, like walking or swimming.

Developing a strong midsection through exercise

Maintaining correct sitting and standing posture

Summary

If the sciatic nerve is pinched or irritated, it can cause sciatica. This can happen, for example, if a disk slips in the spine. Developing muscle strength and flexibility in the affected area can help reduce the likelihood of future damage and expedite the healing process.

A patient and their doctor or physical therapist can work together to determine the best course of treatment, including the most beneficial exercises.